If Lost, Please Contact:

Name:_____

Phone:_____

Dedication

This Intermittent Fasting Book is dedicated to all the enthusiasts out there who want to record their weight loss and diet plan and document their findings in the process.

You are my inspiration for producing books and I'm honored to be a part of keeping all of your intermittent fasting notes and records organized.

This journal notebook will help you record the details of your intermittent fasting.

Thoughtfully put together with these sections to record: Weekly Goals, Exercise Activity, Water Intake, Carbs, Calories, Fasting Hours, Daily Notes, Meals 1 & 2, and Weekly Recap.

How to Use this Book

The purpose of this book is to keep all of your Intermittent Fasting notes all in one place. It will help keep you organized.

This Intermittent Fasting Log will allow you to accurately document every detail about your intermittent fasting.

Here are examples of the prompts for you to fill in and write about your experience in this book:

1. Weekly Goals
2. Exercise Activity
3. Water Intake
4. Carbs
5. Calories
6. Fasting Hours
7. Daily Notes
8. Meals 1 & 2
9. Weekly Recap

A Goal
Without A Plan
Is Just
A Wish

Day 1

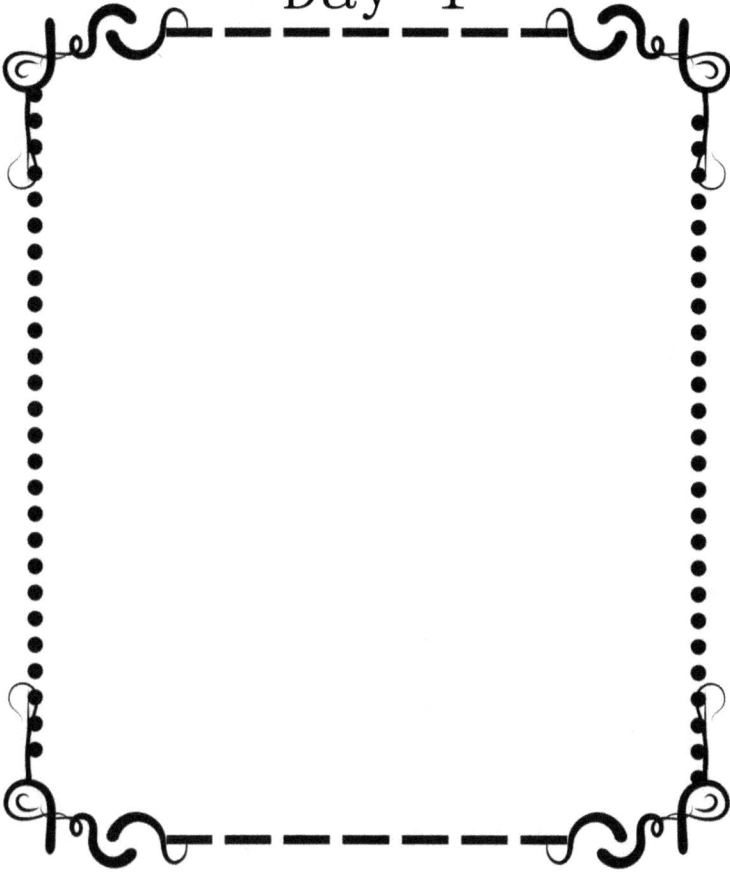

IN THE BEGINNING	
Date	
Weight	
Chest	
Arm	
Waist	
Hips	

Weekly Goals

Daily Fasting Hours:_____

Daily Water Intake:_____

Daily Calories:_____

Daily Carbs:_____

Daily Exercise:_____

My Motivation For The Week

_____
_____
_____
_____
_____
_____
_____
_____
_____
_____
_____
_____

Day 1
Date:

START FAST	END FAST	TOTAL FAST TIME
AM/PM	AM/PM	

Fast Broken With:

_____

Meal 1

Food/Beverage	Cals	Carbs	Fat	Protein
SUBTOTALS				

Meal 2

Food/Beverage	Cals	Carbs	Fat	Protein
SUBTOTALS				

Water Intake

Daily Notes

Day 2

Date:

START FAST AM/PM	END FAST AM/PM	TOTAL FAST TIME

Fast Broken With:

_____

Meal 1

Food/Beverage	Cals	Carbs	Fat	Protein
SUBTOTALS				

Meal 2

Food/Beverage	Cals	Carbs	Fat	Protein
SUBTOTALS				

Water Intake

Daily Notes

_____

_____

_____

_____

_____

_____

_____

_____

_____

_____

_____

_____

_____

_____

_____

_____

_____

_____

_____

Day 3

Date:

START FAST   END FAST   TOTAL FAST TIME
     AM/PM   AM/PM

Fast Broken With:

_____

Meal 1

Food/Beverage	Cals	Carbs	Fat	Protein
SUBTOTALS				

Meal 2

Food/Beverage	Cals	Carbs	Fat	Protein
SUBTOTALS				

Water Intake

Daily Notes

_____
_____
_____
_____
_____
_____
_____
_____
_____
_____
_____
_____
_____
_____
_____
_____
_____
_____
_____
_____
_____

Day 4
Date:

START FAST   END FAST   TOTAL FAST TIME
    AM/PM   AM/PM

Fast Broken With:

_____

Meal 1

Food/Beverage	Cals	Carbs	Fat	Protein
SUBTOTALS				

Meal 2

Food/Beverage	Cals	Carbs	Fat	Protein
SUBTOTALS				

Water Intake

Daily Notes

_____

_____

_____

_____

_____

_____

_____

_____

_____

_____

_____

_____

_____

_____

_____

_____

_____

_____

_____

_____

_____

_____

Day 5
Date:

START FAST   END FAST   TOTAL FAST TIME
     AM/PM   AM/PM

Fast Broken With:

_____

Meal 1

Food/Beverage	Cals	Carbs	Fat	Protein
SUBTOTALS				

Meal 2

Food/Beverage	Cals	Carbs	Fat	Protein
SUBTOTALS				

Water Intake

Daily Notes

_____

_____

_____

_____

_____

_____

_____

_____

_____

_____

_____

_____

_____

_____

_____

_____

_____

_____

Day 6
Date:

START FAST	END FAST	TOTAL FAST TIME
AM/PM	AM/PM	

Fast Broken With:

_____

Meal 1

Food/Beverage	Cals	Carbs	Fat	Protein
SUBTOTALS				

Meal 2

Food/Beverage	Cals	Carbs	Fat	Protein
SUBTOTALS				

Water Intake

Daily Notes

_____

_____

_____

_____

_____

_____

_____

_____

_____

_____

_____

_____

_____

_____

_____

_____

_____

_____

_____

_____

_____

Day 7

Date:

START FAST	END FAST	TOTAL FAST TIME
AM/PM	AM/PM	

Fast Broken With:

_____

Meal 1

Food/Beverage	Cals	Carbs	Fat	Protein
SUBTOTALS				

Meal 2

Food/Beverage	Cals	Carbs	Fat	Protein
SUBTOTALS				

Weekly Recap

Week 1 Success	
Date	
Weight	
Chest	
Arm	
Waist	
Hips	

Daily Fasting Hours Achieved?_____

Daily Water Intake Achieved?_____

Daily Calories Achieved?_____

Daily Carbs Achieved?_____

Daily Exercise Achieved?_____

Struggles This Week

_____

_____

_____

_____

Successes This Week

_____

_____

_____

_____

Notes

_____

_____

_____

_____

_____

_____

_____

_____

_____

_____

_____

_____

_____

_____

_____

_____

_____

_____

Weekly Goals

Daily Fasting Hours:_____

Daily Water Intake:_____

Daily Calories:_____

Daily Carbs:_____

Daily Exercise:

My Motivation For The Week

_____
_____
_____
_____
_____
_____
_____
_____
_____
_____
_____

Day 8
Date:

START FAST   END FAST   TOTAL FAST TIME
   AM/PM   AM/PM

Fast Broken With:

_____

Meal 1

Food/Beverage	Cals	Carbs	Fat	Protein
SUBTOTALS				

Meal 2

Food/Beverage	Cals	Carbs	Fat	Protein
SUBTOTALS				

Water Intake

Daily Notes

_____

_____

_____

_____

_____

_____

_____

_____

_____

_____

_____

_____

_____

_____

_____

_____

_____

_____

_____

Day 9
Date:

START FAST _____ END FAST _____ TOTAL FAST TIME
AM/PM   AM/PM

Fast Broken With:
_____

Meal 1

Food/Beverage	Cals	Carbs	Fat	Protein
SUBTOTALS				

Meal 2

Food/Beverage	Cals	Carbs	Fat	Protein
SUBTOTALS				

Water Intake

Daily Notes

Day 10

Date:

Fast Broken With:

_____

Meal 1

Food/Beverage	Cals	Carbs	Fat	Protein
SUBTOTALS				

Meal 2

Food/Beverage	Cals	Carbs	Fat	Protein
SUBTOTALS				

Water Intake

Daily Notes

_____

_____

_____

_____

_____

_____

_____

_____

_____

_____

_____

_____

_____

_____

_____

_____

_____

_____

_____

_____

_____

Day 11

Date:

START FAST _____ AM/PM   END FAST _____ AM/PM   TOTAL FAST TIME

Fast Broken With:

_____

Meal 1

Food/Beverage	Cals	Carbs	Fat	Protein
SUBTOTALS				

Meal 2

Food/Beverage	Cals	Carbs	Fat	Protein
SUBTOTALS				

Water Intake

Daily Notes

Day 12

Date:

START FAST	END FAST	TOTAL FAST TIME
AM/PM	AM/PM	

Fast Broken With:

_____

Meal 1

Food/Beverage	Cals	Carbs	Fat	Protein
SUBTOTALS				

Meal 2

Food/Beverage	Cals	Carbs	Fat	Protein
SUBTOTALS				

Water Intake

Daily Notes

Day 13

Date:

START FAST   END FAST   TOTAL FAST TIME
      AM/PM   AM/PM

Fast Broken With:

_____

Meal 1

Food/Beverage	Cals	Carbs	Fat	Protein
SUBTOTALS				

Meal 2

Food/Beverage	Cals	Carbs	Fat	Protein
SUBTOTALS				

Water Intake

Daily Notes

_____

_____

_____

_____

_____

_____

_____

_____

_____

_____

_____

_____

_____

_____

_____

_____

_____

_____

_____

_____

Day 14
Date:

START FAST   END FAST   TOTAL FAST TIME
AM/PM   AM/PM

Fast Broken With:

_____

Meal 1

Food/Beverage	Cals	Carbs	Fat	Protein
SUBTOTALS				

Meal 2

Food/Beverage	Cals	Carbs	Fat	Protein
SUBTOTALS				

Water Intake

Daily Notes

_____

_____

_____

_____

_____

_____

_____

_____

_____

_____

_____

_____

_____

_____

_____

_____

_____

_____

_____

_____

_____

Weekly Recap

Week 2 Success

Date

Weight

Chest

Arm

Waist

Hips

Daily Fasting Hours Achieved?_____

Daily Water Intake Achieved?_____

Daily Calories Achieved?_____

Daily Carbs Achieved?_____

Daily Exercise Achieved?_____

Struggles This Week

_____

_____

_____

_____

Successes This Week

_____

_____

_____

_____

Notes

_____

_____

_____

_____

_____

_____

_____

_____

_____

_____

_____

_____

_____

_____

_____

_____

_____

_____

Weekly Goals

Daily Fasting Hours:_____

Daily Water Intake:_____

Daily Calories:_____

Daily Carbs:_____

Daily Exercise:

My Motivation For The Week

_____
_____
_____
_____
_____
_____
_____
_____
_____
_____
_____
_____
_____

Day 15
Date:

START FAST AM/PM	END FAST AM/PM	TOTAL FAST TIME

Fast Broken With:

_____

Meal 1

Food/Beverage	Cals	Carbs	Fat	Protein
SUBTOTALS				

Meal 2

Food/Beverage	Cals	Carbs	Fat	Protein
SUBTOTALS				

Water Intake

Daily Notes

_____

_____

_____

_____

_____

_____

_____

_____

_____

_____

_____

_____

_____

_____

_____

_____

_____

_____

_____

_____

_____

Day 16
Date:

START FAST AM/PM	END FAST AM/PM	TOTAL FAST TIME

Fast Broken With:

_____

Meal 1

Food/Beverage	Cals	Carbs	Fat	Protein
SUBTOTALS				

Meal 2

Food/Beverage	Cals	Carbs	Fat	Protein
SUBTOTALS				

Water Intake

Daily Notes

_____

_____

_____

_____

_____

_____

_____

_____

_____

_____

_____

_____

_____

_____

_____

_____

_____

_____

_____

_____

_____

_____

Day 17

Date:

START FAST	END FAST	TOTAL FAST TIME
AM/PM	AM/PM	

Fast Broken With:

_____

Meal 1

Food/Beverage	Cals	Carbs	Fat	Protein
SUBTOTALS				

Meal 2

Food/Beverage	Cals	Carbs	Fat	Protein
SUBTOTALS				

Water Intake

Daily Notes

_____
_____
_____
_____
_____
_____
_____
_____
_____
_____
_____
_____
_____
_____
_____
_____
_____
_____
_____
_____
_____
_____

Day 18

Date:

START FAST	END FAST	TOTAL FAST TIME
AM/PM	AM/PM	

Fast Broken With:

_____

Meal 1

Food/Beverage	Cals	Carbs	Fat	Protein
SUBTOTALS				

Meal 2

Food/Beverage	Cals	Carbs	Fat	Protein
SUBTOTALS				

Water Intake

Daily Notes

_____

_____

_____

_____

_____

_____

_____

_____

_____

_____

_____

_____

_____

_____

_____

_____

_____

_____

_____

_____

Day 19

Date:

START FAST	END FAST	TOTAL FAST TIME
AM/PM	AM/PM	

Fast Broken With:

_____

Meal 1

Food/Beverage	Cals	Carbs	Fat	Protein
SUBTOTALS				

Meal 2

Food/Beverage	Cals	Carbs	Fat	Protein
SUBTOTALS				

Water Intake

Daily Notes

_____

_____

_____

_____

_____

_____

_____

_____

_____

_____

_____

_____

_____

_____

_____

_____

_____

_____

_____

_____

_____

_____

Day 20
Date:

START FAST	END FAST	TOTAL FAST TIME
AM/PM	AM/PM	

Fast Broken With:

_____

Meal 1

Food/Beverage	Cals	Carbs	Fat	Protein
SUBTOTALS				

Meal 2

Food/Beverage	Cals	Carbs	Fat	Protein
SUBTOTALS				

Water Intake

Daily Notes

_____

_____

_____

_____

_____

_____

_____

_____

_____

_____

_____

_____

_____

_____

_____

_____

_____

_____

_____

_____

_____

_____

Day 21

Date:

START FAST	END FAST	TOTAL FAST TIME
AM/PM	AM/PM	

Fast Broken With:

_____

Meal 1

Food/Beverage	Cals	Carbs	Fat	Protein
SUBTOTALS				

Meal 2

Food/Beverage	Cals	Carbs	Fat	Protein
SUBTOTALS				

Water Intake

Daily Notes

_____

_____

_____

_____

_____

_____

_____

_____

_____

_____

_____

_____

_____

_____

_____

_____

_____

_____

_____

_____

_____

Weekly Recap

	Week 3 Success
Date	
Weight	
Chest	
Arm	
Waist	
Hips	

Daily Fasting Hours Achieved?_____

Daily Water Intake Achieved?_____

Daily Calories Achieved?_____

Daily Carbs Achieved?_____

Daily Exercise Achieved?_____

Struggles This Week

_____

_____

_____

_____

Successes This Week

_____

_____

_____

_____

Notes

_____

_____

_____

_____

_____

_____

_____

_____

_____

_____

_____

_____

_____

_____

_____

_____

_____

_____

Weekly Goals

Daily Fasting Hours:_____

Daily Water Intake:_____

Daily Calories:_____

Daily Carbs:_____

Daily Exercise:_____

My Motivation For The Week

_____

_____

_____

_____

_____

_____

_____

_____

_____

_____

Day 22

Date:

START FAST
AM/PM

END FAST
AM/PM

TOTAL FAST TIME

Fast Broken With:

_____

Meal 1

Food/Beverage	Cals	Carbs	Fat	Protein
SUBTOTALS				

Meal 2

Food/Beverage	Cals	Carbs	Fat	Protein
SUBTOTALS				

Water Intake

Daily Notes

_____
_____
_____
_____
_____
_____
_____
_____
_____
_____
_____
_____
_____
_____
_____
_____
_____
_____
_____

Day 23
Date:

START FAST   END FAST   TOTAL FAST TIME

    AM/PM   AM/PM

Fast Broken With:

_____

Meal 1

Food/Beverage	Cals	Carbs	Fat	Protein
SUBTOTALS				

Meal 2

Food/Beverage	Cals	Carbs	Fat	Protein
SUBTOTALS				

Water Intake

Daily Notes

_____

_____

_____

_____

_____

_____

_____

_____

_____

_____

_____

_____

_____

_____

_____

_____

_____

_____

Day 24

Date:

START FAST   END FAST   TOTAL FAST TIME

     AM/PM   AM/PM

Fast Broken With:

_____

Meal 1

Food/Beverage	Cals	Carbs	Fat	Protein
SUBTOTALS				

Meal 2

Food/Beverage	Cals	Carbs	Fat	Protein
SUBTOTALS				

Water Intake

Daily Notes

_____

_____

_____

_____

_____

_____

_____

_____

_____

_____

_____

_____

_____

_____

_____

_____

_____

_____

_____

_____

_____

Day 25

Date:

Fast Broken With:

_____

Meal 1

Food/Beverage	Cals	Carbs	Fat	Protein
SUBTOTALS				

Meal 2

Food/Beverage	Cals	Carbs	Fat	Protein
SUBTOTALS				

Water Intake

Daily Notes

_____
_____
_____
_____
_____
_____
_____
_____
_____
_____
_____
_____
_____
_____
_____
_____
_____
_____
_____

Day 26

Date:

START FAST
AM/PM

END FAST
AM/PM

TOTAL FAST TIME

Fast Broken With:

_____

Meal 1

Food/Beverage	Cals	Carbs	Fat	Protein
SUBTOTALS				

Meal 2

Food/Beverage	Cals	Carbs	Fat	Protein
SUBTOTALS				

Water Intake

Daily Notes

_____
_____
_____
_____
_____
_____
_____
_____
_____
_____
_____
_____
_____
_____
_____
_____
_____
_____
_____
_____

Day 27
Date:

START FAST	END FAST	TOTAL FAST TIME
AM/PM	AM/PM	

Fast Broken With:
_____

Meal 1

Food/Beverage	Cals	Carbs	Fat	Protein
SUBTOTALS				

Meal 2

Food/Beverage	Cals	Carbs	Fat	Protein
SUBTOTALS				

Water Intake

Daily Notes

_____

_____

_____

_____

_____

_____

_____

_____

_____

_____

_____

_____

_____

_____

_____

_____

_____

_____

_____

_____

Day 28

Date:

Fast Broken With:

_____

Meal 1

Food/Beverage	Cals	Carbs	Fat	Protein
SUBTOTALS				

Meal 2

Food/Beverage	Cals	Carbs	Fat	Protein
SUBTOTALS				

Water Intake

Daily Notes

_____

_____

_____

_____

_____

_____

_____

_____

_____

_____

_____

_____

_____

_____

_____

_____

_____

_____

_____

_____

Weekly Recap

Week 3 Success

Date

Weight

Chest

Arm

Waist

Hips

Daily Fasting Hours Achieved?_____

Daily Water Intake Achieved?_____

Daily Calories Achieved?_____

Daily Carbs Achieved?_____

Daily Exercise Achieved?_____

Struggles This Week

_____

_____

_____

_____

Successes This Week

Notes

Weekly Goals

Daily Fasting Hours:_____

Daily Water Intake:_____

Daily Calories:_____

Daily Carbs:_____

Daily Exercise:

My Motivation For The Week

_____
_____
_____
_____
_____
_____
_____
_____
_____
_____
_____
_____

Day 29

Date:

START FAST	END FAST	TOTAL FAST TIME
AM/PM	AM/PM	

Fast Broken With:

_____

Meal 1

Food/Beverage	Cals	Carbs	Fat	Protein
SUBTOTALS				

Meal 2

Food/Beverage	Cals	Carbs	Fat	Protein
SUBTOTALS				

Water Intake

Daily Notes

_____

_____

_____

_____

_____

_____

_____

_____

_____

_____

_____

_____

_____

_____

_____

_____

_____

_____

_____

_____

_____

_____

Day 30

Date:

START FAST AM/PM	END FAST AM/PM	TOTAL FAST TIME

Fast Broken With:

_____

Meal 1

Food/Beverage	Cals	Carbs	Fat	Protein
SUBTOTALS				

Meal 2

Food/Beverage	Cals	Carbs	Fat	Protein
SUBTOTALS				

Water Intake

Daily Notes

_____

_____

_____

_____

_____

_____

_____

_____

_____

_____

_____

_____

_____

_____

_____

_____

_____

_____

_____

_____

_____

_____

Day 31
Date:

START FAST	END FAST	TOTAL FAST TIME
AM/PM	AM/PM	

Fast Broken With:

_____

Meal 1

Food/Beverage	Cals	Carbs	Fat	Protein
SUBTOTALS				

Meal 2

Food/Beverage	Cals	Carbs	Fat	Protein
SUBTOTALS				

Water Intake

Daily Notes

_____

_____

_____

_____

_____

_____

_____

_____

_____

_____

_____

_____

_____

_____

_____

_____

_____

_____

_____

_____

_____

_____

Monthly Recap

Monthly Success

Date	
Weight	
Chest	
Arm	
Waist	
Hips	

Daily Fasting Hours Achieved?_____

Daily Water Intake Achieved?_____

Daily Calories Achieved?_____

Daily Carbs Achieved?_____

Daily Exercise Achieved?_____

Struggles This Month

_____

_____

_____

_____

Successes This Month

Notes

Day 30

A BEAUTIFUL ENDING	
Date	
Weight	
Chest	
Arm	
Waist	
Hips	

Journal

Journal

Journal

Journal

Journal

Journal

Journal

Journal

Journal

Journal

www.ingramcontent.com/pod-product-compliance
Lightning Source LLC
Chambersburg PA
CBHW051035030426
42336CB00015B/2889